Gout Relief Now!

Your Quick Guide to Gout Treatment, Diet, Medicine, and Home Remedies

David Richards

David Richards

© 2014 Healthy Wealthy nWise Press

All Rights Reserved. No part of this publication may be reproduced in any form or by any means, including scanning, photocopying, or otherwise without prior written permission of the copyright holder.

Disclaimer and Terms of Use: The Author and Publisher has strived to be as accurate and complete as possible in the creation of this book, notwithstanding the fact that she does not warrant or represent at any time that the contents within are accurate due to the rapidly changing nature of the Internet. While all attempts have been made to verify information provided in this publication, the Author and Publisher assumes no responsibility for errors, omissions, or contrary interpretation of the subject matter herein. Any perceived slights of specific persons, peoples, or organizations are unintentional. In practical advice books, like anything else in life, there are no guarantees of income made. This book is not intended for use as a source of legal, business, accounting or financial advice. All readers are advised to seek services of competent professionals in legal, business, accounting, and finance field.

Printed in the United States of America

Table of Contents

INTRODUCTION	6
WHAT EXACTLY IS GOUT?	7
What is Acute Gout? The Painful Truth...	7
The Pain of Gout is Real	8
What Causes Gout Attacks?	8
Warning Signs of Pending Gout Attacks	9
The Symptoms and Complications	9
Gout Complications	10
What is Hyperuricemia?	11
WHO IS PRONE TO GOUT?	11
The Odds of Developing Gout	11
Diseases Which Can Cause a Gout Attack	12
Who is at Risk?	13
TYPES OF GOUT	14
Stages of Idiopathic Gout	14
When to Seek Medical Treatment	15
The Diagnosis of Gout	15
MODERN MEDICAL TREATMENT OF GOUT	17
What is the Best Gout Treatment?	17
Standard Gout Treatment	17
Prevention of Gout	18
HOME REMEDIES GOUT	19
Organic Apple Cider Vinegar	19
Cherries	20
Water	20
Lemon	20
Bananas	21
Ginger Root	21
Herbal Teas	22
Cucumber	22
Garlic	22
Herbs and Spices to Relieve the Pain of Gout	24
Rosemary	24
Red Pepper Flakes	24

Skullcap	*24*
Turmeric	*25*
Mustard	*25*
Charcoal	*25*

THE GOUT DIET — 27

RECIPES TO REDUCE THE INFLAMMATION — 31

SOUPS — 31
- *Basil Red Pepper Soup* — *31*
- *Vegetable Stew* — *32*
- *Gazpacho* — *34*
- *Vegetable Soup* — *35*

ANTI-INFLAMMATORY SALADS — 36
- *Herbed Veggie Pasta Salad* — *36*
- *Mixed Herb Salad with Toasted Seeds* — *37*
- *Citrus Watercress Salad* — *38*
- *Gingery Fruit Salad* — *39*
- *Taco Salad* — *40*
- *Salsa* — *40*
- *Cole Slaw* — *41*

SALAD DRESSINGS — 42
- *Citrus Dressing* — *42*
- *Tomato-Basil Vinaigrette* — *42*

LOW PURINE MAIN DISHES — 43
- *Noodles with Parmesan Cheese Sauce* — *43*
- *Herbed Chicken Breasts* — *44*
- *Sweet Potato Fries* — *45*
- *Italian Beef and Pasta* — *46*

GOUT RELIEF IN A GLASS — 47
- *Fruity Carrot Juice* — *47*
- *Cranberry Tonic* — *47*
- *Ruby Red Delight* — *48*
- *Savory Gout Reliever Juice* — *48*

SAMPLE MENU — 49
SNACKS! — 50
DESSERTS! — 50

EXERCISE AND GOUT! — 51

PAMPER YOURSELF! — 52

RELAXATION TIPS — 52

PAMPERING FOOT SOAKS	53
Epsom Salt Foot Bath	*53*
Ginger Root Poultice	*53*
Mustard Poultice	*53*
Vinegar and Garlic Poultice	*53*
Oil of Elder	*54*
Baking Soda Anti-inflammatory	*54*
CONCLUSION	**55**
CHECK OUT THE OTHER BOOKS IN THE *NATURAL HEALTH & NATURAL CURES SERIES*	**56**
HELPFUL LINKS!	**58**
GLOSSARY	**59**

Introduction

I want to thank you and congratulate you for downloading the book, ***Gout Relief: Your Quick Guide to Gout Treatment, Diet, Medicine, and Home Remedies***.

This book contains proven steps and strategies on how to treat Gout and get the relief you need.

If you are reading this gout guide either you are or someone you love has or is experiencing gout. When it comes to gout the best remedy is educating yourself about gout. You need to know how to what gout is, how to treat it, and how to prevent it. You will want to keep this guide close by it is full of excellent tips, guidance and recipes for gout relief.

Thanks again for downloading this book, I hope you enjoy it!

David Richards

What Exactly is Gout?

Imagine for a minute what it would be like to have a liquid turn into glass in your body and the glass shatters... that is exactly what happens when uric acid changes from liquid form into tiny crystals in your bloodstream. These nasty little crystals like to take up residence in your big toe, stabbing it endlessly with sharp little spears. Sounds like fun, right? This is called gout it's very real and the pain can be unbearable. Even a light blanket can cause horrible pain.

Gout-just the word brings images of red, throbbing, swollen big toes to my mind. You may have experienced this form of arthritis before, but what is Gout? Gout is the most painful form of arthritis, it often occurs in the one of your big toes, especially in the early stages. Gout doesn't develop overnight, it's a condition caused by Acute Gout the buildup of uric acid crystals which collect in the joints and tissues after a number of years.

Uric Acid generally dissolves in the blood stream, but if there is a remarkable increase of uric acid, the kidneys are unable to rid the body of the excess uric acid. If you eat too many foods containing purine the acid levels in the blood become high causing hyperuricemia. Purines are substances which can be found in your body's tissues, when the purines break down uric acid is formed.

What is Acute Gout? The Painful Truth...

Acute Gout is usually defined by:

1. Sudden onset of severe pain and tenderness in a joint, usually the left big toe.

2. Redness and swelling of the tissues, sometimes the tissue is purplish in color.
3. Joint is hot to the touch.
4. Light pressure on the joint causes intense pain.
5. Joints feel stiff when you move them.

The Pain of Gout is Real

The fact is gout pain is very real. The pain of gout can be agony for the sufferer. Some experience only one attack and never have that pain again, they are the lucky ones. While others can have reoccurring attacks, some as soon as one month apart, until the pain and the condition becomes severe.

If you leave the condition untreated, gout can damage your joints. The uric crystals of gout can also move to other areas of your body if left untreated. This can become further debilitating.

What Causes Gout Attacks?

Normally uric acid will dissolve in the blood stream, it then passes through the kidneys and leaves the body in the urine. Sometimes uric acid will build up when:

1. The body increases the amount of uric acid it makes.
2. The kidneys cannot get rid of enough uric acid, if the levels are too high.
3. You eat foods rich in purines.

Foods high in proteins, our lifestyle and our state of health can increase the amounts of purines in our body.

Gout Relief Now!

1. Organ meats, such as liver, sweetbread, and kidney
2. Fish, which includes herrings, mackerel, sardines, mussels and seafood
3. Too much alcohol
4. Drinking beverages high in sugar and fructose. Drinking two or more drinks high in sugar can increase the risk of developing gout by 85%, this can include certain fruit juices and fruits which are high in fructose.
5. Not getting enough Vitamin C
6. Medications such as aspirin, diuretics, and some chemotherapy drugs can increase the levels of uric acid in your body.
7. Some people who have certain conditions such as psoriasis, chronic kidney disease, high blood pressure and hypothyroidism.

Warning Signs of Pending Gout Attacks

The Symptoms and Complications

Gout attacks can slowly develop over the course of one day, it commonly occurs in a toe joint, such as the big toe. They can cause extreme pain, making walking and sleeping difficult, just a small touch from your sheet can produce intense pain. The skin around your big toe may swell, become inflamed and red. The most common time for gout attacks seems to be the nighttime. What are the symptoms of gout?

Extreme pain in a joint-the pain may occur in your hands, wrists, knees, ankles, or feet. The most prevalent joint where the pain occurs is the big toe. The pain can include a hot or warm feeling to the skin as the tissue becomes inflamed.

When the gout attack lessens often you will see some flaking and itching of the skin surrounding the joint.
Often the skin around the tissue around the joint can become red or purplish in color.

Nodules can occur in the ears, hands or elbows.

Some people experience a fever during a gout attack.

The joint becomes less mobile and stiff making it difficult and painful when you move it.

Gout attacks can reoccur within days, weeks, months, or even years later from the original attack.

Gout Complications

If you develop a fever, have intense swelling, pain and redness, your joint may indicate an infection. A visit to your medical professional is important to avoid an advanced infection in the area of the gout.

Stones can form in your kidneys when urate collects in the urinary tract leading to the formation of kidney stones.

If the gout goes untreated the joint can become inflamed, nodules can occur and the joints can become damaged.

Untreated gout has been known to spread to other joints.

What is Hyperuricemia?

Hyperuricemia is a high level of uric acid in the blood. Approximately 2/3 of the total body urate is produced for no apparent reason. 70% of the urate is excreted by the kidneys the rest is eliminated by the intestines. A healthy body weight is important in the prevention of gout. Yet, rapid weight loss can be detrimental because it can increase the uric acid levels in your blood causing hyperuricemia.

Who is Prone to Gout?

People who are unable to efficiently eliminate uric acid through their urine are more likely to develop gout.

The Odds of Developing Gout

1. Did you know that men are more likely to develop gout? Yes, they are more than 4 times as likely to develop gout over women. Women do get gout, but the percentage is low.
2. If your parents had gout sometime in their lifetime, you are 20% more apt to develop gout.
3. If you drink alcohol, your increased alcohol intake, especially beer can increase your chances of having a gout attack.
4. Red meat, liver, heart, kidneys, fish consumption is rich in purines, which can become uric acid crystals if the uric

acid crystals lodge in one or more joints, the result is gout.

Extreme situations can cause gout attacks, and these situations are:

1. Consumption and over-indulgence of organ meats, red meats, sardines, mussel's, and some seafood's.
2. Trauma to a joint
3. Extreme diets
4. Dehydration
5. Chemotherapy treatments
6. Some medications such as, aspirin, nicotinic acid, diuretics, high blood pressure medications, clorosporin A, and allopurinal and probenecid (odd- because these medications are suppose to prevent gout attacks.). Also the vitamin supplement niacin can precipitate an attack.
7. Have an enzyme defect that makes it hard for your body to break down purines.
8. Had an organ transplant
9. Exposure to Occupational Lead

Diseases Which Can Cause a Gout Attack

Diseases and a compromised immune system can be the underlying cause of gout, these diseases and conditions include:

1. Leukemia
2. Lymphoma
3. Chronic Kidney Disease
4. Psoriasis
5. Hypothyroidism
6. Hemoglobin disorders
7. Cancer

8. Allergies
9. Arthritis

Who is at Risk?

Anyone who consumes a Standard American Diet of red meat, mounds of potatoes, rich gravies, biscuits slathered with butter and a large wedge of chocolate layer cake with fudge frosting, is at risk for the inflammation and pain of Gout. Add other bad habits and you may become a victim of Gout. These factors are:

1. Smoking- when a person smokes they release large amounts of free radicals, which produce inflammation in tissues and joints.
2. Excess weight- Adults who are overweight with high levels of inflammatory chemicals in their blood contributes to the risk of developing gout.
3. Sedentary lifestyle- Being a couch potato can increase your chances of experiencing the fire of gout. Exercise helps to balance your body chemistry. It keeps your muscles, and joint flexible, and strengthens them. Exercise actually reduces the inflammation of gout.
4. Stress- When you are stressed it can alter your internal chemistry, and adrenaline and cortisol (stress hormones) deplete our DHEA, which is a natural inflammatory chemical.

Types of Gout

There are three types of gout which can be diagnosed by a medical professional. The three types of gout are:

1. Idiopathic Gout-99% of gout sufferers have this primary form of gout, idiopathic means its origin/cause is unknown. Idiopathic gout comes in three stages, yet not everyone will develop all three stages, some may experience one stage while others will go through two or three stages.
2. Secondary Gout-this gout is the result of taking certain medications, health or disease conditions which can precipitate an attack.
3. Pseudo-gout- Pseudo means fake or imagined gout, some people believe they have gout when actually they are experiencing a calcium buildup in the body, not uric acid.

Stages of Idiopathic Gout

1. Asymptomatic Hyperuricemia- This is the first stage of gout, usually you are free of symptoms, this stage of gout is diagnosed when your blood levels are tests by your medical professional and high levels of uric acid show up in your blood test.

2. Acute Gout Arthritis-If you experience this stage you will know it, this is the painful, inflamed, swollen stage of gout. You begin to believe that your joint is being stabbed by tiny little spears, it's so painful.

3. Interval Phase- This is the stage where you believe your gout is gone, you are free of pain, walking, sleeping, and wearing shoes is no longer filled with intense pain. This is the time where you look for help, to prevent a return of

a gout attack. This is the time to change your diet, to stop smoking, to give up alcohol and strive for a healthy lifestyle. A-h-h-h relief, well for awhile anyway, gout can reoccur if you don't make changes to prevent a return.

4. Chronic Tophaceous Gout- This is the stage of gout no one wants to reach, this is the stage where monosodium urate crystals develop, also called topi. These tophi collect in your joints, bones and cartilage and form pointed clusters which can actually poke through your skin.

When to Seek Medical Treatment

Go to see your medical profession if you experience the following symptoms:

1. Within the span of one day your joint becomes swollen, red, hot and extremely painful.
2. The joint becomes stiff, tight and shiny.
3. You develop a fever, chills, and loss of appetite.
4. You have had this attack more than once.
5. You notice white chalky bumps forming on the joint.

If you ignore these symptoms, you could develop crippling from lack of medical attention.

The Diagnosis of Gout

If you are experiencing the symptoms of gout, your medical professional will take your medical history, ask about your symptoms and if you have a family history of gout (gout is more common if you have family members who have experienced it in the past.)

To confirm a diagnosis of gout your medical professional may draw a sample of fluid from the inflamed joint to look for the uric acid crystals common in gout. This test is called **Arthrocentesis**. This is one of the most reliable tests to determine if your inflammation is gout or not.

Often your medical professional may order **x-rays** of your inflamed joint, looking for *tophi* on your joints.

Blood tests- used to see if there are uric acid levels in your bloodstream.
Urine tests- used to detect uric acid are also known as **Uricosuria**.

These tests are not painful and can answer your question- "Is this gout?" Going untreated is not only painful, but it can also be detrimental to your health.

Modern Medical Treatment of Gout

What is the Best Gout Treatment?

There are many treatments available for gout relief, there are home remedies, the Ayruveda way, homeopathic remedies and then of course the modern traditional methods.

Standard Gout Treatment

Doctors use medication to treat gout attacks, the typical medications are:

1. Nonsteroidal anti-inflammatory drugs (NSAIDs)- these medications include ibuprofen and naproxen which help to manage pain and inflamed joints. Yet these medications have a risk for abdominal pain, bleeding or ulcers in people who take higher dosages of these medications.

2. Colchicines-this medication is meant to knock out the pain of the gout attack. People who are unable to take NASIDs are prescribed Colchicines, yet this medication comes with side effects which includes nausea, vomiting and diarrhea.

3. Steroids-A doctor will give you a steroid shot or in pill form when the gout pain is relentless. Steroids do work well when managing pain, especially for those who are unable to take colchicines and NSAIDs.

4. Uloric-This medication is effective in lowering uric acid levels found in the blood. This medication is known to lower uric acid and relieve chronic gout symptoms.

Prevention of Gout

1. Allopurinol- This popular medication decreases the level of uric acid produced in the blood, decreasing the incidents of developing reoccurring gout attacks. The side effects of this drug are skin rashes and a lowered blood count.
2. Probenecid- This medication assists the kidneys in removing uric acid from your system. Probenecid also helps to prevent further gout attacks. The side effects of this drug are a skin rash, abdominal pains and kidney stones.

Sometimes the side effects can cause greater harm than the relief you may receive, also these medications can become less effective with time. If you want to prevent, instead of medically treat gout then you should consider the natural remedies available today.

Home Remedies Gout

Gout can be treated at home with some simple household remedies and a diet low in purines. These remedies are quite effective in treating all the variations of gout. The following most effective remedies are:

Organic Apple Cider Vinegar

Apple Cider Vinegar helps to treat gout and arthritis. The acidity of apple cider vinegar will help relieve the acute pain. When you add honey to the apple cider vinegar the combination will boost the body's anti-inflammatory response. Apple cider vinegar is beneficial in many ways:

- Apple cider vinegar is rich in enzymes & potassium
- Supports a healthy immune system
- Helps control weight
- Promotes digestion & pH balance
- Helps soothe dry throats
- Helps remove body sludge toxins

Ways to get the benefits of Apple Cider Vinegar:

Mix one teaspoon organic apple cider vinegar in a glass of water and drink it 2 to 3 times daily. If you find this remedy to be effective, you may increase the dosage of apple cider vinegar up to 2 tablespoons.

Another remedy is to mix 2 tablespoons of organic apple cider vinegar with two tablespoons of honey. Take this combination 2 times daily once in the morning and once before going to bed.

Cherries

Cherries have been noted to relieve the symptoms of gout there are several ways to consume cherries for their benefits.

Eat about 15 sweet raw cherries per day to obtain optimal relief from gout attacks.

Drink cherry juice-one whole glass of cherry juice at least once per day is very beneficial to get relief from the symptoms of gout.

Take 1 tablespoon of cherry concentrate 3 times per day.

Black, sweet, yellow and sour cherries all were effective in reducing the inflammation and pain of gout. Cherries are rich in Vitamin C which helps in eliminating the gout deposits in your joints

Water

Water is one of the best remedies to prevent and relieve gout pain. Drink 6-8 ounce glasses of water a day. Water flushes out the urate crystals and uric acid from our body through urination. Drinking water will keep your kidneys flushed out to prevent the formation of kidney stones.

Lemon

Lemon juice helps to alkalize your body by neutralizing the uric acid in your system. Lemon is rich in Vitamin C, which will help in dissolving uric acid crystals and deposits, relieving the inflammation and pain of gout. Lemon juice also helps to strengthen the body tissues which prevent gout attacks.

Squeeze the juice of one lemon in a glass of water. Drink this juice three times a day, morning, noon and night. Lemon juice is one of the most effective home remedies available. It really works!

Increasing the intake of citrus fruits, berries, tomatoes, green peppers and leafy green vegetables have a high Vitamin C content. Vitamin C helps to reduce the inflammation of gout. Eating these raw fruits and vegetables is the best diet for gout sufferers.

Bananas

Bananas serve as a good remedy for preventing gout. You will need to consume 3-4 bananas a day. Bananas are rich in phosphorus and potassium which can chemically react with the uric acid crystals and help to eliminate them from your body.

Ginger Root

Ginger has anti-inflammatory properties which reduce the pain and inflammation common in gout.

Mix equal amounts of fenugreek powder, turmeric powder and dried ginger. Mix one teaspoon of this mixture in one cup warm water and drink it twice a day.

Add ginger root in cooking recipes, you can also eat a small raw piece of ginger root daily.

You may add ½ teaspoon of ginger to one cup of boiling water, mix well and drink it once a day.

Herbal Teas

Another way to increase your intake of liquids is to drink herbal teas. Coffee, regular teas, cocoa and colas have caffeine which can increase the likelihood of developing gout. Herbal teas come in handy little pouches which makes tea brewing easy to access. When you drink Chamomile tea two to three times a day it works wonders to relieve the symptoms of gout.

Cucumber

Cucumber removes the fluid which can build up in your tissues due to the increase of uric acid. Cucumber will relieve the swelling and fluid buildup which collects in your gouty joint.

Take a few slices of peeled cucumber and place in one cup of boiling water, let steep for at least 20 minutes and drink it often throughout the day.

Garlic

Garlic has a substance called *allicin* which helps to reduce inflammations. It is best to take the garlic as raw fresh garlic for the best results. There are garlic capsules available, but they aren't as affective as the fresh garlic is.

Herbs and Spices to Relieve the Pain of Gout

Herbs and spices have a soothing affect when applied as a paste or ointment to the inflamed gouty joint.

Rosemary

Rosemary is a great antioxidant, and this potion will relieve the inflammation of gout when used as a local pain reliever.

Take a handful of rosemary and chop it finely, add the rosemary to a pint of olive oil and allow it to sit for one week. After the mixture has had a chance to blend, strain the rosemary from the olive oil, store the oil in a cool dry place and use in cooking and in salads.

Red Pepper Flakes

Capsaicin is the ingredient in red pepper flakes which help to reduce or block the pain signals to the brain, which relieves the symptoms of gout. Using red pepper flakes in your cooking is all you need to reduce the pain of gout. Capsaicin now comes in a convenient capsule form, when you take one or two capsules three or four times per day, with juice you will enjoy the benefits of red pepper flakes.

Skullcap

It is easier to obtain skullcap in capsule form, even though it grows in many locales. Skullcap reduces inflammation and joint swelling when you take one to two capsules after a fatty meal. For the best results take 3 to 4 capsules once or twice daily to prevent an attack.

Turmeric

This spice has anti-inflammatory benefits and is often an ingredient in most Indian foods. ½ teaspoon of turmeric powder in water or juice twice a day will help most gout sufferers get relief.

Mustard

Mix equal quantities of whole wheat powder and mustard powder and add just enough water to make a paste. Apply on the affected part and leave overnight for relief and get the rest you need.

Charcoal

Charcoal draws toxins out of the body including uric acid. There are three ways to use charcoal.

1. Place a couple of teaspoons of powdered charcoal into a basin of warm to hot water and soak your affected joint for 30 minutes. This will soothe the aching joint, giving you the pain relief you want now.

2. Mix several teaspoonfuls of powdered charcoal with an equal amount of flaxseeds with warm water to make a paste, apply this paste to your gouty joint then cover with a cloth or piece of plastic, change the charcoal paste every four hours to obtain pain relief.

3. Activated charcoal comes in capsule form take the capsules 3-4 times a day for best results. It is wise to ask your medical professional about this remedy, some people cannot take activated charcoal capsules, due to other health conditions.

The Gout Diet

Diet plays an important role in regulating the uric acid levels in your blood.

Eating a healthy nutritious diet low in purine's goes a long way to prevent or relieve gout attacks. These foods contain potassium, iron complex carbohydrates and are low in proteins and purines. Here are some tips and foods which will decrease or eliminate uric acid buildup.

Eat light foods, preferably steamed or boiled. Enjoy whole grain breads and cereals.

Increase Vitamin C intake, eat citrus fruit, tomatoes, green peppers, strawberries often during the day.

Avoid eggs, organ meat and red meat. In fact, avoid all foods which are high uric acid producing especially foods high in protein.

Avoid white flour, fried and processed foods.

Salmon and chicken can be eaten sparingly.

Drink plenty of water to keep well hydrated and, to keep the uric acid diluted and to flush it out with your urine.

Avoid caffeine, soda drinks, tea, coffee, alcohol and beer.

Avoid eating large amounts of peas, lentils, beans, mushrooms, oats and yeast products.

An apple a day, actually two apples a day after a meal keeps the gout away. Apples contain *Malic acid* which neutralizes uric acid.

Try to stay away from fried foods, and fast foods, having them as a treat occasionally is okay just not every day, unless you want a return of your gout.

Increase your consumption of Omega-3 fatty acids, they will reduce inflammation. Omega-3 fatty acid rich foods include flax seeds, walnuts and mercury free tuna.

For desserts stick with fresh fruits or low-fat, low-sugar sherbets.

Foods High in Purines- Avoid

Hearts and other organ meats
Herrings
Mussels
Yeast
Smelt
Sardines
Meat Broths
Meat Gravies
Crab
Red Meats

Foods Moderately High in Purines

Anchovies
Mutton
Veal
Bacon (Sorry)
Liver
Turkey
Kidneys
Trout

Goose
Haddock
Scallops

Good Foods to Eat

Eat foods in the low glycemic index such as brown rice, squash, and apples,

Enjoy the following vegetables without fear of increasing your uric acid levels:

Beets
Broccoli
Brussels sprouts
Cabbage
Carrots
Celery
Cucumbers
Green beans
Squash
Leafy greens such as lettuce, spinach, mustard greens, especially kale
Radishes
Red, yellow and green bell peppers
Sprouts of all kinds such as bean, alfalfa, mung bean sprouts, and sprouted grains
Turnips

Avoiding foods high in purines is the best way to avoid gout attacks. Avoiding or eating small amounts of red meats, organ meats, lamb, mackerel, shrimp, lobster and scallops, will help prevent reoccurrences of gout. Keep servings of meat, chicken and fish to 2-3 ounces per serving. Drink plenty of water to help flush out the uric acid in your system. Water is one of the best "medicines" when it comes to preventing gout. 6-8 glasses of water with a little lemon insures good health and a better quality of life.

Eat less fats-Saturated fats reduces your body's ability to excrete uric acid, cause you to gain weight and increases your risk factors to develop gout.

Avoid alcohol- Beer and alcoholic drinks interrupt the body's excretion of uric acid. This is especially true if you are experiencing a gout attack.

High fructose foods-We all love our sweets, but they should be eaten in moderation. Juices and soft drinks should be avoided due to the fact that high fructose can increase the production of uric acid. Pure, whole, 100% fruit juice is the way to go to prevent an attack.

Complex carbohydrates- Whole grain breads, vegetables, and fruit are the perfect food for people who suffer from gout. Avoid refined sugar treats such as candy, cakes and doughnuts.

Recipes to Reduce the Inflammation

Soups

Basil Red Pepper Soup

I love this soup it has a beautiful rich red color and makes a delightful light lunch perfect when paired with a yummy green salad.

5 large red bell peppers, seeded, cut in 1 inch pieces
3 cloves of garlic, coarsely chopped
2 1/2 cups water
¼ cup (packed) fresh basil leaves, chopped
1 teaspoon apple cider vinegar
1 tablespoon extra-virgin olive oil
Salt and black pepper to taste

1. Combine red peppers, garlic and water in a medium saucepan. Bring to boil then reduce heat to low. Cover and simmer until tender, about 25 minutes.

2. Transfer red peppers and garlic to food processor, reserving cooking liquid. Process until smooth, adding cooking liquid as needed to reach desired consistency. Discard extra cooking liquid.

3. Return soup to pan and heat to serving temperature. Stir in basil, vinegar, olive oil and salt and pepper. Serve and enjoy!

David Richards

Vegetable Stew

This hearty stew is rib-sticking good, yet soothing and will help to reduce the inflammation of gout, due to the plentiful anti-oxidants.

2 tablespoons olive oil
3 cups minced onion
3 medium cloves garlic, minced
2 medium potatoes, diced
1 medium eggplant, diced
1 teaspoon salt
Black pepper to taste
2 medium stalks celery, chopped
1 stalk broccoli, chopped
2 medium carrots, sliced or diced
2 small zucchini, diced
3 tablespoons tomato paste
3 tablespoons molasses
2 teaspoons dill
Optional Toppings: Sour cream or yogurt, finely minced parsley

1. Heat oil in a Dutch oven. Add onion, garlic, potatoes, eggplant, salt and pepper. Cover and cook over medium heat, stirring often, until the potatoes are tender.

2. Add small amounts of water, as needed to prevent sticking. Add celery, broccoli and carrots.

3. Continue to cook over medium heat, covered but occasionally stirring, until all the vegetables begin to be tender (8-10 minutes). Add remaining ingredients (except

toppings) and stir. Cover and simmer about 15 minutes more, stirring occasionally.
4. Taste to correct seasonings.

5. Serve piping hot, topped with sour cream or yogurt and minced parsley.

David Richards

Gazpacho

This tomato rich summer soup is delicious anytime of the year.

2 cups tomatoes
3" slice of cucumber
1 bell pepper
2 tbsp onion chopped
1 garlic clove
1 tsp salt
4 tsp extra virgin olive oil
4 tsp apple cider vinegar
1 tsp sugar
3/4 cup water

1. Wash and chop all vegetables. Place chopped vegetables in blender with all liquids. Blend until smooth.

2. Add salt and sugar to taste.

3. Pour into airtight container, seal and refrigerate overnight to infuse flavors.

4. Serve one quarter of the soup as a snack mid-morning and midafternoon.

Gout Relief Now!

Vegetable Soup

Reduce your gouty inflammation and make your stomach happy too! Cayenne is a great anti-inflammatory spice.

4 Tbsp olive oil
1 medium carrot, peeled and chopped into small pieces
1 large onion, chopped
2 cloves garlic, crushed
1 Tbsp. grated fresh ginger
1 large potato, peeled and diced into ½ inch cubes
4 medium tomatoes, chopped
1 cup finely chopped coriander leaves
5 cups water
2 tsp. salt
1 tsp. pepper
1 tsp. cumin
1/8 tsp. cayenne

1. Heat oil in a saucepan, then stir-fry carrots, onion, garlic, and ginger over medium heat for 5 minutes.

2. Add potatoes, tomatoes, and coriander leaves, then stir-fry for an additional 5 minutes.

3. Add remaining ingredients then bring to boil. Cover and simmer over medium low heat for 1 hour or until vegetables are well done, adding more water if necessary.

4. Purée, then return to saucepan and heat before serving.

Anti- Inflammatory Salads

Herbed Veggie Pasta Salad

1/4 cup extra virgin olive oil

1 tablespoon tarragon vinegar

1 teaspoon basil

1/4 teaspoon garlic

1/4 tablespoon pepper

1/4 teaspoon dried dill weed

3 cups cooked pasta shells

1 zucchini, sliced thinly

1/3 cup radishes - sliced thinly

2 1/4 carrots - sliced thin

2 3/4 tablespoons green onion – chopped

1. In blender or a food processor, combine oil, vinegar, basil, garlic, pepper and dill weed to make the dressing.
2. Put remainder of ingredients in a bowl and toss.
3. Pour dressing over salad and toss once more. Serve.

Mixed Herb Salad with Toasted Seeds

This delicious light salad is packed with anti-inflammatory agents, which helps to relieve the pain and swelling associated with gout. Fresh parsley contains vitamin C and iron, while the pumpkin seeds and sunflower seeds are filled with vitamins, minerals, including vitamin E, iron and zinc.

4 cups of mixed salad greens
2 cups mixed salad herbs (coriander, parsley, basil and arugula)
3 tablespoons pumpkin seeds
3 tablespoons sunflower seeds

Dressing
4 tablespoons extra virgin olive oil
1 tablespoon balsamic vinegar
½ teaspoon Dijon mustard
Salt and pepper to taste

1. For the dressing, whisk the ingredients with a fork in a small bowl or in a screw top jar and shake well.

2. Place the salad greens and herbs in a large bowl.

3. Toast the pumpkin and sunflower seeds in a fry pan for 2 minutes or until golden brown, toss frequently to prevent burning. Cool slightly then sprinkle over the salad.

4. Pour the dressing over the salad and toss gently until the leaves are well coated with dressing. Serve.

David Richards

Citrus Watercress Salad

Watercress is a peppery, slightly bitter green which goes wonderful with sweet sour flavor of the citrus fruit. You may substitute arugula and endive if watercress isn't available in your area. Citrus fruit helps to lower uric acid levels in your body.

1 large orange peeled and sectioned
1 grapefruit peeled and sectioned
1 lime peeled and sectioned
1 tablespoon extra-virgin olive oil
2 cloves of garlic
¼ teaspoon pepper
Salt to taste
4 cups watercress

Dressing:

1. Combine ¼ of orange, ¼ of grapefruit with the lime, oil garlic, pepper and salt, mash fruit slightly with fork to release the citrus juices and mixing ingredients well.

2. Place watercress and remaining citrus fruit in a large bowl.

3. Pour dressing over the watercress and toss lightly to cover the leaves completely. Enjoy!

Gout Relief Now!

Gingery Fruit Salad

Try this fruity, refreshing salad which is packed with antioxidants plus the benefits of vitamin A and the anti-inflammatory agents of ginger.

1 cup cubed cantaloupe
1 papaya, peeled, seeded and cubed
2 kiwifruit, peeled, and sliced
1 cup fresh pineapple chunks
1 lime, peeled and sectioned
½ teaspoon grated fresh gingerroot
1 tablespoon chopped fresh mint leaves

Combine all the ingredients, tossing gently. Serve.

David Richards

Taco Salad

4 chicken breasts (boiled)
1 large yellow onion (diced)
1 can black olives
1 15 oz can tomatoes with green chilies
1 head iceberg lettuce
Shredded low-fat cheddar cheese
Chili powder
Cumin
2 tbsp olive oil
Low-fat sour cream
Guacamole

1. Shred the chicken with a fork
2. Heat olive oil in skillet over medium
3. Sautee' one quarter of the onions
4. Add chicken, cumin, chili powder and tomatoes
5. Simmer for 20 minutes, stirring occasionally
6. While mixture is simmering, shred lettuce and place in bowls olives, sour cream and onions and guacamole.

Serve with salsa.

Salsa

1 large peeled tomato and sliced
1 small bunch cilantro
1 medium onion
Garlic salt to taste

Combine ingredients in blender. Serve over taco salad.

Cole Slaw

1 cup shredded cabbage
2 tbsp mayonnaise
2 tsp white distilled vinegar
Salt and black pepper to taste

Mix ingredients. Add salt and pepper to taste.

David Richards

Salad Dressings

Citrus Dressing

1 orange juiced
2 Tablespoons lemon juice
1 Tablespoon balsamic vinegar
1 clove garlic pressed
¼ teaspoon sea salt
¼ teaspoon dry mustard
½ teaspoon Stevia

Whisk all ingredients until well mixed or shake in a jar. Serve as a salad dressing.

Tomato-Basil Vinaigrette

½ cup olive oil
1/3 cup apple cider vinegar
¼ cup raw honey
3 tablespoons chopped fresh basil
2 cloves garlic, minced
Sea salt to taste

Whisk ingredients in a bowl and serve.

Low Purine Main Dishes

Noodles with Parmesan Cheese Sauce

This is a delicious low purine noodle dish.

1 lb thin noodles
1 cup grated parmesan cheese
2 crushed cloves garlic
4 tbsp finely chopped fresh coriander
6 tbsp olive oil
Salt and black pepper to taste

1. Place noodles in pot of boiling water for 11 minutes or until cooked.
2. Drain noodles and place in bowl.
3. Stir remaining ingredients into noodles and serve while warm.

David Richards

Herbed Chicken Breasts

Even though meat is usually a no-no when you have gout, you may have it in small amounts, approximately 3 oz per meal (about the size of a deck of cards) is allowed.

1 pound boneless, skinless chicken breast
2 teaspoons olive oil
Olive oil cooking spray
1 tablespoon lemon juice
½ teaspoon rosemary
¼ teaspoon salt
¼ teaspoon black pepper

1. Brush chicken breasts lightly with olive oil and place in a baking pan which has been coated with olive oil cooking spray.
2. Drizzle with lemon juice and sprinkle remaining ingredients evenly over chicken pieces.
3. Bake at 400° for 15 to 20 minutes or until tender and the juices are clear. Broil for 1 minute to lightly brown chicken if desired.

Excellent with Sweet Potato Fries!

Gout Relief Now!

Sweet Potato Fries

These delicious sweet potato fries are baked not deep fried and very tasty! The cayenne pepper adds the right kick and has an anti-inflammatory agents.

4 sweet potatoes
1 teaspoon olive oil
1/8 cayenne pepper
Salt to taste

1. Preheat oven to 450°. Cut sweet potatoes (unpeeled) lengthwise into ½ inch slices and cut each slice into sticks.
2. Combine oil and cayenne in a large bowl and add sweet potatoes. Toss to coat.
3. Place sweet potatoes in a single layer on a baking sheet. Bake 15 minutes, turn over with a spatula and continue baking until tender another 15 minutes. Sprinkle with salt.

David Richards

Italian Beef and Pasta

½ pound lean hamburger
¼ cup dried minced onion
½ teaspoon dried minced garlic
2 -8 oz cans of no-salt-added tomato sauce
6 oz can tomato paste
1 teaspoon dried Italian seasoning
2 ½ cups water
½ teaspoon salt
1½ cups uncooked corkscrew macaroni
1 cup shredded part-skim Mozzarella cheese

1. Cook hamburger in a large pan over low heat until meat is browned, and crumbled.
2. Add onion, garlic, tomato sauce, tomato paste, Italian seasoning, water and salt. Cover and bring to boil over medium heat, stirring occasionally to prevent sticking.
3. Add pasts, cover and cook for 15 to 18 minutes or until pasta is done. Stir occasionally after adding pasta.
4. Remove from heat. Top with shredded cheese.

Gout Relief in a Glass

Fruity Carrot Juice

Cut up and mix in your juicer:

4 carrots
1 ounce of fresh strawberries
1 slice of pineapple
1 mango
1 lime
1 small cucumber

Drink this morning and afternoon. It helps to prevent gout attacks and lessen the painful swelling.

Cranberry Tonic

Mix together 1 quart of cold water and 1 ounce of fresh cranberries.

Bring mixture to a boil and heat for 3 minutes.

Strain and chill.

Drinking three glasses daily will help your body get rid of excess uric acid.

David Richards

Ruby Red Delight

Beets are phytonutrient rich and an excellent anti-inflammatory.

½ inch piece of ginger peeled
2 oranges peeled
4 oz beets (3 small)

Juice produce as follows: ginger, oranges, and beets. Stir well and serve over ice.

Savory Gout Reliever Juice

A savory juice filled with anti-inflammatory properties

Use your juicer to juice the following:
5 stalks of celery
A handful of parsley
2 carrots
1 clove garlic
2 inch piece of ginger
1 cup of filtered water

You can drink this juice on a regular basis once a day.

Sample Menu

Breakfast:

½ cup orange juice
½ cup farina
Strawberries
Whole grain toast with jelly and 1 teaspoon margarine
1 cup 2% milk
Coffee

Lunch:

Hamburger on a bun (3oz)
Sweet Potato Fries
Apple
2% milk

Dinner:

1 **Herbed Chicken Breast** (3 oz)
Tossed Salad with **Tomato Basil** Vinaigrette
½ cup rice
½ cup broccoli
Dinner roll with 1 teaspoon margarine
½ cup sherbet
Iced tea

Snacks!

We love our snacks, when on a low purine diet you need to choose your items carefully. Good choices are: fresh fruit, vegetables with a low fat dip or cottage cheese, celery, crackers or toast with peanut butter. Portion control is important, so don't overdo the snacks, but enjoy small amounts between meals to avoid overeating during meal times. Remember drink plenty of fluids to keep uric acid levels down!

Desserts!

Desserts are the perfect ending to our meals and they keep us full longer. The best dessert of course is fresh fruit! Fruit is low in purines, so you can consume as much as you desire without the fear of having a gout attack. Also gelatins, ice milk, vanilla wafers, angel food cake, and low-fat frozen yogurts are desserts you can enjoy. Within reason.

Exercise and Gout!

Moderate exercise is beneficial to maintain flexibility, good range of motion and strengthen your joints. Jogging and endurance exercises can stress your joints, so it is to be avoided.

Swimming and exercising in a swimming pool is a great way to exercise, it can also help to relieve gouty joints, increase your strength and gets your blood flowing.

Bicycling, walking, and water aerobics, are appropriate exercises for gout suffers. They keep your muscles and joints flexible and strong.

Exercise is a good habit to have, make it a part of your everyday lifestyle, whether you suffer from gout or not. Your body needs to exercise to remain healthy and strong, and it makes you feel good.

There is no cure for gout, but you can prevent gout attacks by eating a healthy diet, low in purines, drink plenty of liquids-water during the day, try one of the home remedies before or if you have a gout attack, exercise and take care of yourself.

Stress, worry and forgetting to take care of you can bring on a gout attack. You deserve to take care of your body, to remain healthy and pain free. Begin doing it now!

Pamper Yourself!

When you have a gout attack fasting is a great way to pamper yourself. Give your system and yourself a rest for good results. Getting rid of the toxins in your body will benefit you in many ways, besides treating the gout.

When you have an acute attack, drink just orange juice and water for 3 days. After the symptoms lessen take an all fruit diet for next 3 days. Thereafter, take fresh fruits, sprouts and raw vegetables.

No canned, refined, processed and fried foods during this fast.

When you are having an attack don't stand for long periods of time. Standing adds pressure to the painful joint causing more pain. Put your feet up on a pillow and relax.

Relaxation Tips

Rest and relax
Listen to your favorite serene music
Take up Yoga
Mediate
Take a bubble bath
Read a good book
Think positive thoughts
Take a slow walk in the park or wooded area, enjoy nature
Smile more often, it releases endorphins in your brain
Take good care of you!

Pampering Foot Soaks

Epsom Salt Foot Bath

To 1 gallon of hot water add 2 cups of Epsom salt and 1 cup of vinegar. Keep the affected foot dipped in this soak for 20 minutes. It removes the swelling and pain extremely fast.

Ginger Root Poultice

Another use for ginger is making a paste of ginger root with a little water and then apply the paste to the affected joint.

Mustard Poultice

Mix equal quantities of whole wheat powder and mustard powder and add just enough water to make a paste. Apply on the affected part and leave overnight for relief and get the rest you need.

Vinegar and Garlic Poultice

Mix 1 tablespoon vinegar, 1 tablespoon Wheat Bran and 2 crushed garlic cloves. Use this mixture as a poultice on your swollen joint.

Oil of Elder

Soak a cotton ball in oil of elder and apply to the painful joint.

Baking Soda Anti-inflammatory

Make a paste of baking soda and water. Apply to the affected areas as an anti-inflammatory agent.

Conclusion

Thank you again for downloading this book!

I hope it was able to help you to get the gout relief you need and find the remedies to be helpful, gout can hamper our quality of life, don't suffer anymore!

The next step is to take action to prevent the reoccurrence of gout attacks.

Finally, if you enjoyed this book, please take the time to share your thoughts and post a review on Amazon. It'd be greatly appreciated!

Thank you and good luck!

David Richards

Check out the other books in the Natural Health & Natural Cures Series

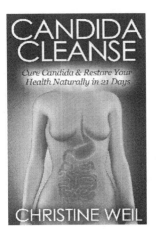

http://www.amazon.com/dp/B00IIRQH9K

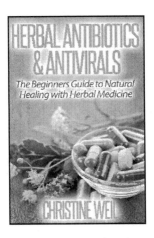

https://www.amazon.com/dp/B00J2F1QDO

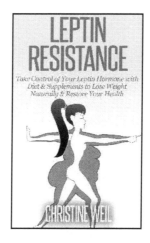

http://www.amazon.com/dp/B00J8UNBWW

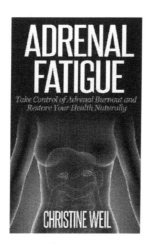

http://www.amazon.com/dp/B00J8SHS6E

Helpful Links!

www.ihatemygout.com

www.niams.nih.gov

www.ayurvedaininstitute.org

www.blissplan.com/homeremedies

www.gout-aware.com

www.backwoodshome.com

Glossary

Arthritis- inflammation of the joints

Diuretics- agents that increase urine secretion

Gout- Gout is the most painful form of arthritis, it often occurs in the one of your big toes, especially in the early stages. Gout doesn't develop overnight, it's a condition caused by Acute Gout the buildup of uric acid crystals which collect in the joints and tissues after a number of years.

Uric Acid generally dissolves in the blood stream, but if there is a remarkable increase of uric acid, the kidneys are unable to rid the body of the excess uric acid. If you eat too many foods containing purine the acid levels in the blood become high causing hyperuricemia.

Hyperuricemia- is a high level of uric acid in the blood. Approximately 2/3 of the total body urate is produced for no apparent reason. 70% of the urate is excreted by the kidneys the rest is eliminated by the intestines. A healthy body weight is important in the prevention of gout. Yet, rapid weight loss can be detrimental because it can increase the uric acid levels in your blood causing hyperuricemia.

Inflammation- a bodily response to injury or disease in which heat, redness and swelling are present

Kidney Disease- gout is a progressive chronic disease that can damage the kidneys.

Nodules- a small roundish lump or mass

Purines- are substances which can be found in your body's tissues, when the purines break down uric acid is formed

Made in the USA
Lexington, KY
12 April 2015